Super-Easy Vegan Keto Dishes for Busy People

Super-fast Plant-Based Ketogenic Recipes to Create your Tasty and Healthy Meals

Karen Yosco

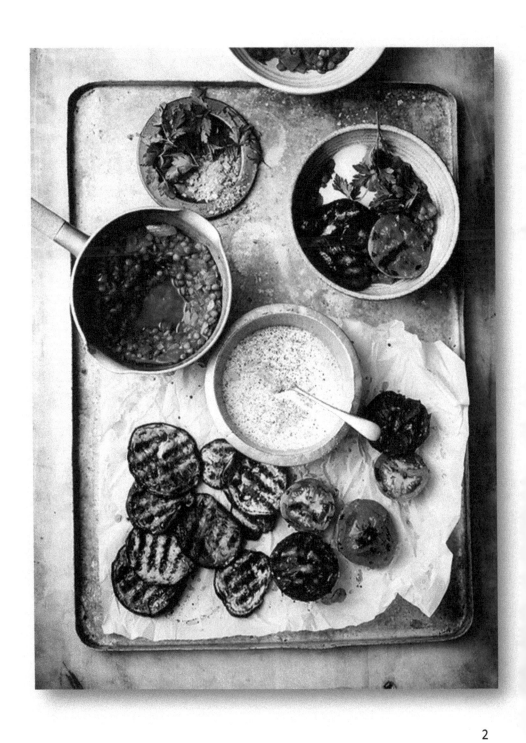

By reading this document, the reader agrees that under no circumstances is the author responsible for any losses, direct or indirect, which are incurred as a result of the use of information contained within this document, including, but not limited to, — errors, omissions, or inaccuracies.

Table of Contents

BREAKFAST 8

Chocolate and Hazelnut Smoothie 8

Blueberry Oatmeal Smoothie 10

Orange French Toast 12

LUNCH...14

Veggie Noodles...14

Minutes Vegetarian Pasta 16

Pesto Quinoa with White Beans 18

DINNER 20

Spicy Carrots and Olives 20

Tamarind Avocado Bowls 22

Avocado and Leeks Mix 24

Cabbage Bowls 26

Pomegranate and Pears Salad............................... 28

Bulgur and Tomato Mix 30

Beans Mix 32

STIR-FRIED, GRILLED VEGETABLES................... 34

Grilled Seitan with Creole Sauce 34

Mushroom Steaks..37

DIP AND SPREAD RECIPES 40

Chunky Cucumber Salsa....................................... 40

Low-fat Stuffed Mushrooms 42

PASTA & NOODLES 44

Vegetable Penne Pasta... 44

SIDE DISHES *46*

Pinto Bean Stew with Cauliflower *46*

Tempeh White Bean Gravy *49*

Broccoli and Black Bean Chili *51*

SOUP AND STEW *53*

Mushroom & Broccoli Soup *53*

Creamy Cauliflower Pakora Soup *55*

Garden Vegetable and Herb Soup *57*

The Mediterranean Delight with Fresh Vinaigrette *59*

Moroccan Vegetable Stew *61*

Red Lentil Soup *64*

SMOOTHIES AND BEVERAGES *66*

Simple Date Shake *66*

BREAD RECIPES *68*

Mashed Potato Bread *68*

Healthy Celery Loaf *70*

Broccoli and Cauliflower Bread *72*

SAUCES, DRESSINGS, AND DIPS *74*

Avocado-dill Dressing *74*

SALADS RECIPES *76*

Sweet Potato & Black Bean Protein Salad *76*

FRUIT SALAD RECIPES *79*

Asian Fruit Salad *79*

ENTRÉES *81*

Chickpea Avocado Salad Sandwiches *81*

GRAINS AND BEANS *83*

Veggie Paella *83*

Spiced Tomato Brown Rice.. 85

DRINKS...87

Strawberry Pink Drink 87

Almond Butter Brownies 89

Quick Chocó Brownie.. 91

Coconut Peanut Butter Fudge 92

DESSERTS 94

Cashew-Chocolate Truffles.. 94

Banana Chocolate Cupcakes 96

Minty Fruit Salad... 98

Cherry-Vanilla Rice Pudding (Pressure cooker) 100

OTHER RECIPES 102

Delicious Lentil Soup...102

Trail Mix...104

Flax Crackers 105

BREAKFAST

Chocolate and Hazelnut Smoothie

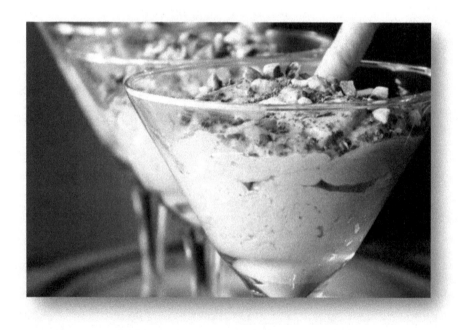

Preparation Time: 5 minutes

Cooking Time: 0 minutes

Servings: 4

Ingredients:

- 1 frozen banana

- 1 cup hazelnuts, unsalted, roasted

- 8 teaspoons maple syrup

- 4 tablespoons cocoa powder, unsweetened

- 1/2 teaspoon hazelnut extract, unsweetened

- 2 cups almond milk, unsweetened

- 1 cup of ice cubes

Directions:

1. Add all the ingredients in the order into a food processor or blender and then pulse for 1 to 2 minutes until blended, scraping the sides of the container frequently.

2. Distribute the smoothie among glasses and then serve.

Nutrition: 198 Cal 12 g Fat 1 g Saturated Fat 21 g Carbohydrates 5 g Fiber 12 g Sugars 5 g Protein;

Blueberry Oatmeal Smoothie

Preparation Time: 5 minutes

Cooking Time: 0 minutes

Servings: 4

Ingredients:

- 2 cups frozen blueberries
- 1 cup old-fashioned oats
- 2 teaspoons cinnamon
- 2 tablespoons maple syrup
- 1 cup spinach
- 2 cup almond milk, unsweetened
- 8 ice cubes

Directions:

1. Add all the ingredients in the order into a food processor or blender and then pulse for 1 to 2 minutes until blended, scraping the sides of the container frequently.

2. Distribute the smoothie among glasses and then serve.

Nutrition: 194 Cal 5 g Fat 3 g Saturated Fat 34 g Carbohydrates 5 g Fiber 15 g Sugars 5 g Protein

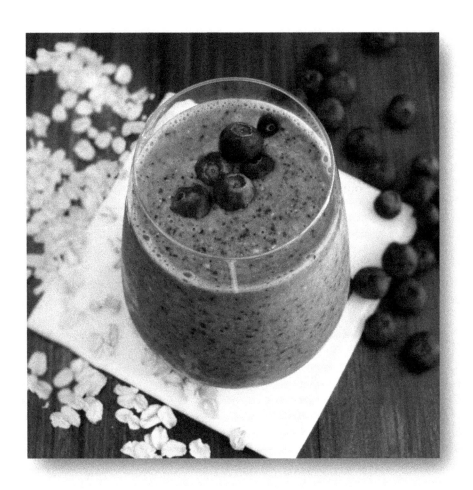

Orange French Toast

Preparation Time: 5 minutes

Cooking Time: 30 minutes

Servings: 8 servings

Ingredients:

- 2 cups of plant milk (unflavored)
- Four tablespoon maple syrup
- 11/2 tablespoon cinnamon
- Salt (optional)
- 1 cup flour (almond)
- 1 tablespoon orange zest
- 8 bread slices

Directions:

1. Turn the oven and heat to 400 degree F afterwards.
2. In a cup, add **Ingredients:** and whisk until the batter is smooth.
3. Dip each piece of bread into the paste and permit to soak for a couple of seconds.

4. Put in the pan, and cook until lightly browned.

5. Put the toast on the cookie sheet and bake for ten to fifteen minutes in the oven, until it is crispy.

Nutrition: Calories: 129 Fat: 1.1g Carbohydrates: 21.5g Protein: 7.9g

LUNCH

Veggie Noodles

Preparation Time: 10 minutes

Cooking Time: 5 minutes

Servings: 2

Ingredients:

- 2 tablespoons vegetable oil

- 4 spring onions, divided

- 1 cup snap pea

- 2 tablespoons brown sugar

- 9 oz. dried rice noodles, cooked

- 5 garlic cloves, minced

- 2 carrots, cut into small sticks

- 3 tablespoons soy sauce

Directions:

1. Heat vegetable oil in a skillet over medium heat and add garlic and 3 spring onions.

2. Cook for about 3 minutes and add the carrots, peas, brown sugar and soy sauce.

3. Add rice noodles and cook for about 2 minutes.

4. Season with salt and black pepper and top with remaining spring onion to serve.

Nutrition: Calories: 25; Fat: 2.0g Protein: 5.2g Carbohydrates: 5.3g Fiber: 4g; Sodium: 18mg

Minutes Vegetarian Pasta

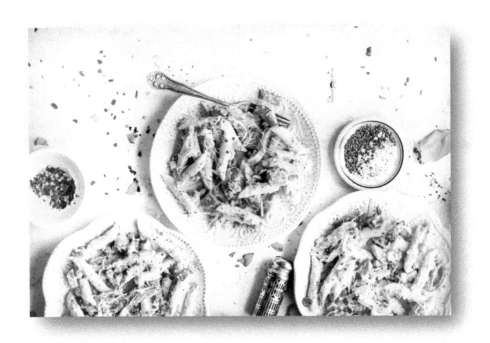

Preparation Time: 5 minutes

Cooking Time: 16 minutes

Servings: 4

Ingredients:

- 3 shallots, chopped

- ¼ teaspoon red pepper flakes

- ¼ cup vegan parmesan cheese

- 2 tablespoons olive oil

- 2 garlic cloves, minced

- 8-ounces spinach leaves

- 8-ounces linguine pasta

- 1 pinch salt

- 1 pinch black pepper

Directions:

1. Boil salted water in a large pot and add pasta.

2. Cook for about 6 minutes and drain the pasta in a colander.

3. Heat olive oil over medium heat in a large skillet and add the shallots.

4. Cook for about 5 minutes until soft and caramelized and stir in the spinach, garlic, red pepper flakes, salt and black pepper.

5. Cook for about 5 minutes and add pasta and 2 ladles of pasta water.

6. Stir in the parmesan cheese and dish out in a bowl to serve.

Nutrition: Calories: 25; Fat: 2.0g Protein: 5.2g Carbohydrates: 5.3g Fiber: 4g; Sodium: 18mg

Pesto Quinoa with White Beans

Preparation Time: 5 minutes

Cooking Time: 15 minutes

Servings: 4

Ingredients:

- 12 ounces cooked white bean

- 3 ½ cups quinoa, cooked

- 1 medium zucchini, sliced

- ¾ cup sun-dried tomato

- ¼ cup pine nuts

- 1 tablespoon olive oil

For the Pesto:

- 1/3 cup walnuts

- 2 cups arugula

- 1 teaspoon minced garlic

- 2 cups basil

- ¾ teaspoon salt

- ¼ teaspoon ground black pepper

- 1 tablespoon lemon juice

- 1/3 cup olive oil

- 2 tablespoons water

Directions:

1. Prepare the pesto, and for this, place all of its ingredients in a food processor and pulse for 2 minutes until smooth, scraping the sides of the container frequently and set aside until required.

2. Take a large skillet pan, place it over medium heat, add oil and when hot, add zucchini and cook for 4 minutes until tender-crisp.

3. Season zucchini with salt and black pepper, cook for 2 minutes until lightly brown, then add tomatoes and white beans and continue cooking for 4 minutes until white beans begin to crisp.

4. Stir in pine nuts, cook for 2 minutes until toasted, then remove the pan from heat and transfer zucchini mixture into a medium bowl.

5. Add quinoa and pesto, stir until well combined, then distribute among four bowls and then serve.

Nutrition: 352 Cal 27.3 g Fat 5 g Saturated Fat 33.7 g Carbohydrates 5.7 g Fiber 4.5 g Sugars 9.7 g Protein

DINNER

Spicy Carrots and Olives

Preparation Time: 15 minutes

Cooking Time: 10 minutes

Servings: 4

Ingredients:

- ½ teaspoon hot paprika

- 1 red chili pepper, minced

- ¼ teaspoon ground cumin

- ¼ teaspoon dried oregano

- ¼ teaspoon dried basil

- ½ teaspoon salt

- 1 tablespoon olive oil

- 1 pound baby carrots, peeled

- 1 cup kalamata olives, pitted and halved

- juice of 1 lime

Directions:

1. Heat up a pan with the oil over medium heat, add the carrots, olives and the other ingredients, toss, cook for 10 minutes, divide between plates and serve.

Nutrition: Calories 141 Fat 5.8 Fiber 4.3 Carbs 7.5 Protein 9.6

Tamarind Avocado Bowls

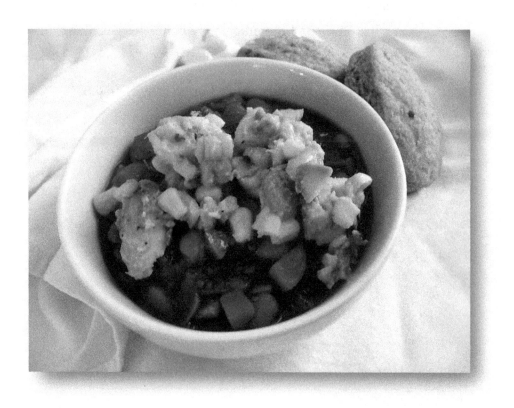

Preparation Time: 10 minutes

Cooking Time: 0 minutes

Servings: 2

Ingredients:

- 1 teaspoon cumin seeds

- 1 tablespoon olive oil

- ½ teaspoon gram masala

- 1 teaspoon ground ginger

- 2 avocados, peeled, pitted and roughly cubed

- 1 mango, peeled, and cubed

- 1 cup cherry tomatoes, halved

- ½ teaspoon cayenne pepper

- 1 teaspoon turmeric powder

- 3 tablespoons tamarind paste

Directions:

1. In a bowl, mix the avocados with the mango and the other ingredients, toss and serve.

Nutrition: Calories 170 Fat 4.5 Fiber 3 Carbs 5 Protein 6

Avocado and Leeks Mix

Preparation Time: 10 minutes

Cooking Time: 0 minutes

Servings: 4

Ingredients:

- 1 small red onion, chopped
- 2 avocados, pitted, peeled and chopped
- 1 teaspoon chili powder
- 2 leeks, sliced
- 1 cup cucumber, cubed
- 1 cup cherry tomatoes, halved
- Salt and black pepper to the taste
- 2 tablespoons cumin powder
- 2 tablespoons lime juice
- 1 tablespoon parsley, chopped

Directions:

1. In a bowl, mix the onion with the avocados, chili powder and the other ingredients, toss and serve.

Nutrition: Calories 120 Fat 2 Fiber 2 Carbs 7 Protein 4

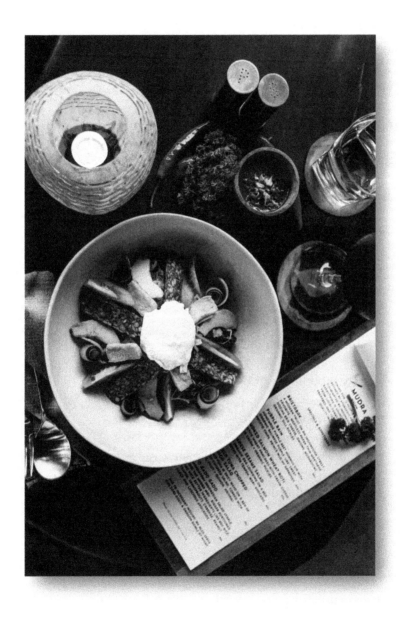

Cabbage Bowls

Preparation Time: 10 minutes

Cooking Time: 10 minutes

Servings: 4

Ingredients:

- 1 green cabbage head, shredded
- 1 red cabbage head, shredded
- 1 teaspoon garam masala
- 1 teaspoon basil, dried
- 1 teaspoon coriander, ground
- 1 teaspoon mustard seeds
- 1 tablespoon balsamic vinegar
- ¼ cup tomatoes, crushed
- A pinch of salt and black pepper
- 3 carrots, shredded
- 1 yellow bell pepper, chopped
- 1 orange bell pepper, chopped

- 1 red bell pepper, chopped

- 2 tablespoons dill, chopped

- 2 tablespoons olive oil

Directions:

1. Heat up a pan with the oil over medium heat, add the peppers and carrots and cook for 2 minutes.

2. Add the cabbage and the other ingredients, toss, cook for 10 minutes, divide between plates and serve.

Nutrition: Calories 150 Fat 9 Fiber 4 Carbs 3.3 Protein 4.4

Pomegranate and Pears Salad

Preparation Time: 10 minutes

Cooking Time: 0 minutes

Servings: 3

Ingredients:

- 3 big pears, cored and cut with a spiralizer

- ¾ cup pomegranate seeds

- 2 cups baby spinach

- ½ cup black olives, pitted and cubed

- ¾ cup walnuts, chopped1 tablespoon olive oil

- 1 tablespoon coconut sugar

- 1 teaspoon white sesame seeds

- 2 tablespoons chives, chopped

- 1 tablespoon balsamic vinegar

- 1 garlic clove, minced

- A pinch of sea salt and black pepper

Directions:

1. In a bowl, mix the pears with the pomegranate seeds, spinach and the other ingredients, toss and serve.

Nutrition: Calories 200 Fat 3.9 Fiber 4 Carbs 6 Protein 3.3

Bulgur and Tomato Mix

Preparation Time: 15 minutes

Cooking Time: 0 minutes

Servings: 4

Ingredients:

- 1 ½ cups hot water

- 1 cup bulgur

- Juice of 1 lime

- 1 cup cherry tomatoes, halved

- 4 tablespoons cilantro, chopped

- ½ cup cranberries, dried

- juice of ½ lemon

- 1 teaspoon oregano, dried

- 1/3 cup almonds, sliced

- ¼ cup green onions, chopped

- ½ cup red bell peppers, chopped

- ½ cup carrots, grated

- 1 tablespoon avocado oil

- A pinch of sea salt and black pepper

Directions:

1. Place bulgur into a bowl, add boiling water to it, stir, and cover and set aside for 15 minutes.

2. Fluff bulgur with a fork and transfer to a bowl.

3. Add the rest of the ingredients, toss and serve.

Nutrition: Calories 260 Fat 4.4 Fiber 3 Carbs 7 Protein 10

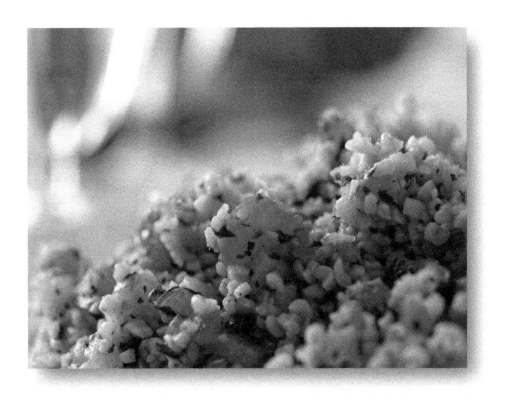

Beans Mix

Preparation Time: 10 minutes

Cooking Time: 15 minutes

Servings: 4

Ingredients:

- 1 ½ cups cooked black beans

- 1 cup cooked red kidney beans

- ½ teaspoon garlic powder

- ½ teaspoon smoked paprika

- 2 teaspoons chili powder

- 1 tablespoon olive oil

- 1 ½ cups chickpeas, cooked

- 1 teaspoon garam masala

- 1 red bell pepper, chopped

- 2 tomatoes, chopped

- 1 cup cashews, chopped

- ½ cup veggie stock

- 1 tablespoon balsamic vinegar

- 1 tablespoon oregano, chopped

- 1 tablespoon dill, chopped

- 1 cup corn kernels, chopped

Directions:

1. Heat up a pan with the oil over medium heat, add the beans, garlic powder, chili powder and the other ingredients, toss and cook for 15 minutes.

2. Divide between plates and serve.

Nutrition: Calories 300 Fat 8.3 Fiber 3.3 Carbs 6 Protein 13

STIR-FRIED, GRILLED VEGETABLES

Grilled Seitan with Creole Sauce

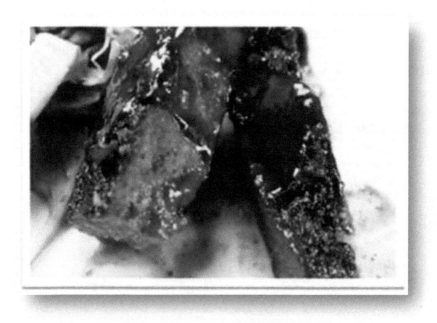

Preparation Time: 10 minutes

Cooking Time: 14 minutes

Servings: 4

Ingredients:

Grilled Seitan Kebabs:

- 4 cups seitan, diced
- 2 medium onions, diced into squares
- 8 bamboo skewers
- 1 can coconut milk
- 2½ tablespoons creole spice
- 2 tablespoons tomato paste
- 2 cloves of garlic

Creole Spice Mix:

- 2 tablespoons paprika
- 12 dried peri chili peppers
- 1 tablespoon salt
- 1 tablespoon freshly ground pepper
- 2 teaspoons dried thyme
- 2 teaspoons dried oregano

Directions:

1. Prepare the creole seasoning by blending all its ingredients and preserve in a sealable jar.

2. Thread seitan and onion on the bamboo skewers in an alternating pattern.

3. On a baking sheet, mix coconut milk with creole seasoning, tomato paste and garlic.

4. Soak the skewers in the milk marinade for 2 hours.

5. Prepare and set up a grill over medium heat.

6. Grill the skewers for 7 minutes per side.

7. Serve.

Nutrition: Calories: 407 Total Fat: 42g Carbs: 13g Net Carbs: 6g Fiber: 1g Protein: 4g

Mushroom Steaks

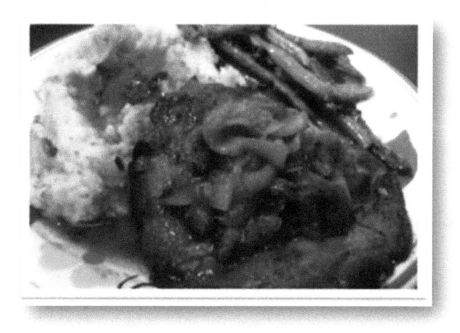

Preparation Time: 10 minutes

Cooking Time: 24 minutes

Servings: 4

Ingredients:

- 1 tablespoon vegan butter

- ½ cup vegetable broth

- ½ small yellow onion, diced

- 1 large garlic clove, minced

- 3 tablespoons balsamic vinegar

- 1 tablespoon mirin

- ½ tablespoon soy sauce

- ½ tablespoon tomato paste

- 1 teaspoon dried thyme

- ½ teaspoon dried basil

- A dash of ground black pepper

- 2 large, whole portobello mushrooms

Directions:

1. Melt butter in a saucepan over medium heat and stir in half of the broth.

2. Bring to a simmer then add garlic and onion. Cook for 8 minutes.

3. Whisk the rest of the ingredients except the mushrooms in a bowl.

4. Add this mixture to the onion in the pan and mix well.

5. Bring this filling to a simmer then remove from the heat.

6. Clean the mushroom caps inside and out and divide the filling between the mushrooms.

7. Place the mushrooms on a baking sheet and top them with remaining sauce and broth.

8. Cover with foil then place it on a grill to smoke.

9. Cover the grill and broil for 16 minutes over indirect heat.

10. Serve warm.

Nutrition: Calories: 887 Total Fat: 93g Carbs: 29g Net Carbs: 13g Fiber: 4g Protein: 8g

DIP AND SPREAD RECIPES

Chunky Cucumber Salsa

Preparation Time: 20 minutes

Cooking Time: 20 minutes

Servings: 4

Ingredients:

- 3 medium cucumbers, peeled and coarsely chopped

- 1 medium mango, coarsely chopped

- 1 cup frozen corn, thawed

- 1 medium sweet red pepper, coarsely chopped

- 1 small red onion, coarsely chopped

- 1 jalapeno pepper, finely chopped

- 3 garlic cloves, minced

- 2 tablespoon white wine vinegar

- 1 tablespoon minced fresh cilantro

- 1 teaspoon salt

- 1/2 teaspoon sugar

- 1/4 to 1/2 teaspoon cayenne pepper

Directions:

1. Mix all ingredients in a big bowl, then chill, covered, about 2 to 3 hours before serving.

Nutrition: Calories 215 Fat 5 Carbs 23 Protein 10

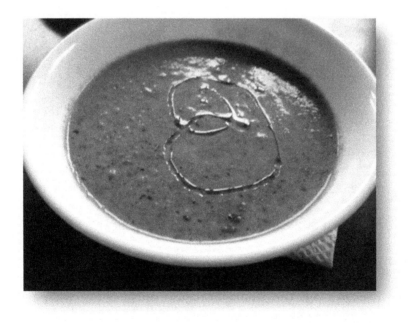

Low-fat Stuffed Mushrooms

Preparation Time: 20 minutes

Cooking Time: 25 minutes

Servings: 6

Ingredients:

- 1 lb. large fresh mushrooms

- 3 tablespoons seasoned bread crumbs

- 3 tablespoons fat-free sour cream

- 2 tablespoons grated Parmesan cheese

- 2 tablespoons minced chives

- 2 tablespoons reduced-fat mayonnaise

- 2 teaspoons balsamic vinegar

- 2 to 3 drops hot pepper sauce, optional

Directions:

1. Take out the stems from the mushrooms, then put the cups aside. Chop the stems and set aside 1/3 cup (get rid of the leftover stems or reserve for later use).

2. Mix the reserved mushroom stems, hot pepper sauce if preferred, vinegar, mayonnaise, chives, Parmesan cheese, sour cream, and breadcrumbs in a bowl, then stir well.

3. Put the mushroom caps on a cooking spray-coated baking tray and stuff it with the crumb mixture.

4. Let it boil for 5 to 7 minutes, placed 4-6 inches from the heat source, or until it turns light brown.

Nutrition: Calories 435 Fat 4 Carbs 23 Protein 9

PASTA & NOODLES

Vegetable Penne Pasta

Preparation Time: 15 minutes

Cooking Time: 20 minutes

Servings: 6

Ingredients:

- ½ large onion, chopped

- 2 celery sticks, chopped

- ½ tablespoon ginger paste

- ½ cup green bell pepper

- 1½ tablespoons soy sauce

- ½ teaspoon parsley

- Salt and black pepper, to taste

- ½ pound penne pasta, cooked

- 2 large carrots, diced

- ½ small leek, chopped

- 1 tablespoon olive oil

- ½ teaspoon garlic paste

- ½ tablespoon Worcester sauce

- ½ teaspoon coriander

- 1 cup water

Directions:

1. Heat olive oil in a wok on medium heat and add onions, garlic and ginger paste.

2. Sauté for about 3 minutes and stir in all bell pepper, celery sticks, carrots and leek.

3. Sauté for about 5 minutes and add remaining ingredients except for pasta.

4. Cover the lid and cook for about 12 minutes.

5. Stir in the cooked pasta and dish out to serve warm.

Nutrition: Calories: 385 Total Fat: 29g Protein: 26g Total Carbs: 5g Fiber: 1g Net Carbs: 4g

SIDE DISHES

Pinto Bean Stew with Cauliflower

Preparation Time: 10 min

Cooking Time: 25 min

Servings: 2

Ingredients:

- 1 cup water

- 1 teaspoon salt

- ¼ cup pinto beans

- 2 tablespoons coconut oil

- ½ small onion chopped

- 1 small zucchini chopped

- ½ teaspoon garlic powder

- 1 bay leaf

- 1 1/2 cups low sodium vegetable stock

- ½ cup steamed cauliflower

- ¼ cup grated mozzarella

- 1 tablespoon chopped fresh cilantro

Directions:

1. In a large bowl, dissolve 1 tablespoon of salt in the water. Add the pinto beans and soak at room temperature for 8 to 24 hours. Drain and rinse.

2. Select Sauté and adjust to Normal or Medium heat. Add the coconut oil to the Instant Pot and heat until shimmering. Add the onion and zucchini, and sprinkle with salt. Cook, stirring often, until the onion pieces separate and soften. Add the garlic powder and cook for about 1 minute, or until fragrant. Add the drained pinto beans, remaining ¼ teaspoon of salt, bay leaf, and vegetable stock.

3. Lock the lid into place. Select Pressure Cook or Manual, and adjust the pressure to High and the time to 15 minutes. After cooking, let the pressure release naturally for 10 minutes, then quick release any remaining pressure.

4. Unlock the lid. Stir in the cauliflower and bring to a simmer to heat it through and thicken the sauce slightly.

Taste the beans and adjust the seasoning. Ladle into bowls and sprinkle with the mozzarella cheese and cilantro.

Nutrition: Calories 245, Total Fat 16. 2g, Saturated Fat 13. 7g, Cholesterol 2mg, Sodium 1745mg, Total Carbohydrate 22. 4g , Dietary Fiber 5.6g , Total Sugars 4. 5g, Protein 7.7g

Tempeh White Bean Gravy

Preparation Time: 05 min

Cooking Time: 20 min

Servings: 2

Ingredients:

- ½ cup cups vegetable broth
- ¼ cup soy sauce
- ¼ cup coconut oil
- 1 teaspoon garlic powder
- ½ cup chopped onion
- 1 cup chopped tempeh
- 1/8 teaspoon dried basil
- 1/8 teaspoon dried parsley
- 1/8 teaspoon ground black pepper
- 1 cup white beans, drained and rinsed
- Enough water

Directions:

1. Add vegetable broth, soy sauce, coconut oil, garlic powder, onion, tempeh, basil, parsley, black pepper and white beans to the Instant Pot. Pour the remaining ¼ cup water over everything.

2. Choose the soup function for 20 minutes.

3. Once done, remove the lid.

4. Serve and enjoy.

Nutrition: Calories 376, Total Fat 29. 4g, Saturated Fat 23. 6g, Cholesterol 0mg, Sodium 2233mg, Total Carbohydrate 22. 4g, Dietary Fiber 4. 9g, Total Sugars 4. 2g, Protein 9. 2g

Broccoli and Black Bean Chili

Preparation Time: 15 min

Cooking Time: 15 min

Servings: 2

Ingredients:

- ½ tablespoon coconut oil
- 1 cup broccoli
- 1 cup chopped red onions
- ½ tablespoon paprika
- 1/2 teaspoon salt
- ¼ cup tomatoes
- 1 cup black beans drained, rinsed
- ¼ chopped green chills
- ½ cup water

Directions:

1. In the Instant Pot, select Sauté; adjust to normal. Heat coconut oil in Instant Pot. Add broccoli, onions, paprika

and salt; cook 8 to 10 minutes, stirring occasionally, until thoroughly cooked. Select Cancel.

2. Stir in tomatoes, black beans, chills and water. Secure lid, set pressure valve to Sealing. Select manual, cook on High pressure 5 minutes. Select Cancel. Keep pressure valve in sealing position to release pressure naturally.

Nutrition: Calories 408, Total Fat 5. 3g, Saturated Fat 3. 4g, Cholesterol 0mg, Sodium 607mg, Total Carbohydrate 70. 7g, Dietary Fiber 18. 1g, Total Sugars 6g, Protein 23. 3g

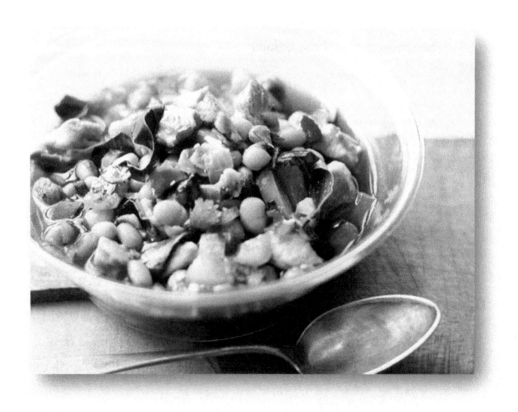

SOUP AND STEW

Mushroom & Broccoli Soup

Preparation Time: 20 minutes

Cooking Time: 45 minutes

Servings: 8

Ingredients:

- 1 bundle broccoli (around 1-1/2 pounds)

- 1 tablespoon canola oil

- 1/2 pound cut crisp mushrooms

- 1 tablespoon diminished sodium soy sauce

- 2 medium carrots, finely slashed

- 2 celery ribs, finely slashed

- 1/4 cup finely slashed onion

- 1 garlic clove, minced

- 1 container (32 ounces) vegetable juices

- 2 cups of water

- 2 tablespoons lemon juice

Directions:

1. Cut broccoli florets into reduced down pieces. Strip and hack stalks.

2. In an enormous pot, heat oil over medium-high warmth; saute mushrooms until delicate, 4-6 minutes. Mix in soy sauce; expel from skillet.

3. In the same container, join broccoli stalks, carrots, celery, onion, garlic, soup, and water; heat to the point of boiling. Diminish heat; stew, revealed, until vegetables are relaxed, 25-30 minutes.

4. Puree soup utilizing a drenching blender. Or then again, cool marginally and puree the soup in a blender; come back to the dish.

5. Mix in florets and mushrooms; heat to the point of boiling. Lessen warmth to medium; cook until broccoli is delicate, 8-10 minutes, blending infrequently. Mix in lemon juice.

Nutrition: Kcal: 830 Carbohydrates: 8 g Protein: 45 g Fat: 64 g

Creamy Cauliflower Pakora Soup

Preparation Time: 20 minutes

Cooking Time: 20 minutes

Servings: 8

Ingredients:

- 1 huge head cauliflower, cut into little florets

- 5 medium potatoes, stripped and diced

- 1 huge onion, diced

- 4 medium carrots, stripped and diced

- 2 celery ribs, diced

- 1 container (32 ounces) vegetable stock

- 1 teaspoon garam masala

- 1 teaspoon garlic powder

- 1 teaspoon ground coriander

- 1 teaspoon ground turmeric

- 1 teaspoon ground cumin

- 1 teaspoon pepper

- 1 teaspoon salt

- 1/2 teaspoon squashed red pepper chips

- Water or extra vegetable stock

- New cilantro leaves

- Lime wedges, discretionary

Directions:

1. In a Dutch stove over medium-high warmth, heat initial 14 fixings to the point of boiling. Cook and mix until vegetables are delicate, around 20 minutes. Expel from heat; cool marginally. Procedure in groups in a blender or nourishment processor until smooth. Modify consistency as wanted with water (or extra stock). Sprinkle with new cilantro. Serve hot, with lime wedges whenever wanted.

2. Stop alternative: Before including cilantro, solidify cooled soup in cooler compartments. To utilize, in part defrost in cooler medium-term.

3. Warmth through in a pan, blending every so often and including a little water if fundamental. Sprinkle with cilantro. Whenever wanted, present with lime wedges.

Nutrition: Kcal: 248 Carbohydrates: 7 g Protein: 1 g Fat: 19 g

Garden Vegetable and Herb Soup

Preparation Time: 20 minutes

Cooking Time: 30 minutes

Servings: 8

Ingredients:

- 2 tablespoons olive oil

- 2 medium onions, hacked

- 2 huge carrots, cut

- 1 pound red potatoes (around 3 medium), cubed

- 2 cups of water

- 1 can (14-1/2 ounces) diced tomatoes in sauce

- 1-1/2 cups vegetable soup

- 1-1/2 teaspoons garlic powder

- 1 teaspoon dried basil

- 1/2 teaspoon salt

- 1/2 teaspoon paprika

- 1/4 teaspoon dill weed

- 1/4 teaspoon pepper

- 1 medium yellow summer squash, split and cut

- 1 medium zucchini, split and cut

Directions:

1. In a huge pan, heat oil over medium warmth. Include onions and carrots; cook and mix until onions are delicate, 4-6 minutes. Include potatoes and cook 2 minutes. Mix in water, tomatoes, juices, and seasonings.

2. Heat to the point of boiling. Diminish heat; stew, revealed, until potatoes and carrots are delicate, 9 minutes.

3. Include yellow squash and zucchini; cook until vegetables are delicate, 9 minutes longer. Serve or, whenever wanted, puree blend in clusters, including extra stock until desired consistency is accomplished.

Nutrition: Kcal: 252 Carbohydrates: 12 g Protein: 1 g Fat: 11 g

The Mediterranean Delight with Fresh Vinaigrette

Preparation Time: 5 minutes

Cooking Time: 10 minutes

Servings: 2

Ingredients:

- Herbed citrus vinaigrette:

- 1 tablespoon of lemon juice

- 2 tablespoons of orange juice

- ½ teaspoon of lemon zest

- ½ teaspoon of orange zest

- 2 tablespoons of olive oil

- 1 tablespoon of finely chopped fresh oregano leaves

- Salt to taste

- Black pepper to taste

- 2-3 tablespoons of freshly julienned mint leaves

- Salad:

- 1 freshly diced medium-sized cucumber

- 2 cups of cooked and rinsed chickpeas

- ½ cup of freshly diced red onion

- 2 freshly diced medium-sized tomatoes

- 1 freshly diced red bell pepper

- ¼ cup of green olives

- ½ cup of pomegranates

Directions:

1. In a large salad bowl, add the juice and zest of both the lemon and the orange along with oregano and olive oil. Whisk together so that they are mixed well. Season the vinaigrette with salt and pepper to taste.

2. After draining the chickpeas, add them to the dressing. Then, add the onions. Give them a thorough mix, so that the onion and chickpeas absorb the flavors.

3. Now, chop the rest of the veggies and start adding them to the salad bowl. Give them a good toss.

4. Lastly, add the olives and fresh mint. Adjust the salt and pepper as required.

5. Serve this Mediterranean delight chilled — a cool summer salad that is good for the tummy and the soul.

Nutrition: Kcal: 286 Carbohydrates: 29 g Protein: 1 g Fat: 11 g

Moroccan Vegetable Stew

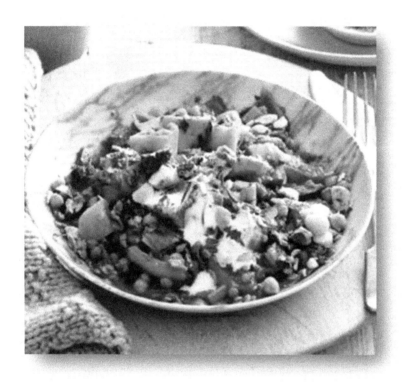

Preparation Time: 5 minutes

Cooking Time: 35 minutes

Servings: 4

Ingredients:

- 1 tablespoon olive oil

- 2 medium yellow onions, chopped

- 2 medium carrots, cut into 1/2-inch dice

- 1/2 teaspoon ground cumin

- 1/2 teaspoon ground cinnamon or allspice

- 1/2 teaspoon ground ginger

- 1/2 teaspoon sweet or smoked paprika

- 1/2 teaspoon saffron or turmeric

- 1 (14.5-ounce) can diced tomatoes, undrained

- 8 ounces green beans, trimmed and cut into 1-inch pieces

- 2 cups peeled, seeded, and diced winter squash

- 1 large russet or other baking potato, peeled and cut into 1/2-inch dice

- 11/2 cups vegetable broth

- 11/2 cups cooked or 1 (15.5-ounce) can chickpeas, drained and rinsed

- ¾ cup frozen peas

- 1/2 cup pitted dried plums (prunes)

- 1 teaspoon lemon zest

- Salt and freshly ground black pepper

- 1/2 cup pitted green olives

- 1 tablespoon minced fresh cilantro or parsley, for garnish

- 1/2 cup toasted slivered almonds, for garnish

Directions:

1. In a large saucepan, heat the oil over medium heat. Add the onions and carrots, cover, and cook for 5 minutes. Stir in the cumin, cinnamon, ginger, paprika, and saffron. Cook, uncovered, stirring, for 30 seconds.

2. Add the tomatoes, green beans, squash, potato, and broth and bring to a boil. Reduce heat to low, cover, and simmer until the vegetables are tender, about 20 minutes.

3. Add the chickpeas, peas, dried plums, and lemon zest. Season with salt and pepper to taste. Stir in the olives and simmer, uncovered, until the flavors are blended, about 10 minutes. Sprinkle with cilantro and almonds and serve immediately.

Nutrition: Calories: 71 kcal Fat: 2.8g Carbs: 9.8g Protein: 3.7g

Red Lentil Soup

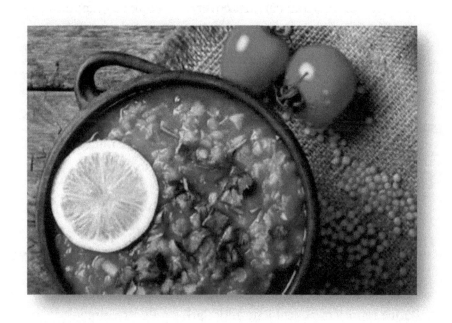

Preparation Time: 5 Minutes

Cooking Time: 25 Minutes

Servings: Makes 6 cups

Ingredients:

- 2 tbsp. Nutritional Yeast

- 1 cup Red Lentil, washed

- ½ tbsp. Garlic, minced

- 4 cups Vegetable Stock

- 1 tsp. Salt

- 2 cups Kale, shredded

- 3 cups Mixed Vegetables

Directions:

1. To start with, place all ingredients needed to make the soup in a large pot.

2. Heat the pot over medium-high heat and bring the mixture to a boil.

3. Once it starts boiling, lower the heat to low. Allow the soup to simmer.

4. Simmer it for 10 to 15 minutes or until cooked.

5. Serve and enjoy.

Nutrition: Calories: 212 kcal Fat: 11.9g Carbs: 31.7g Protein: 7.3g

SMOOTHIES AND BEVERAGES

Simple Date Shake

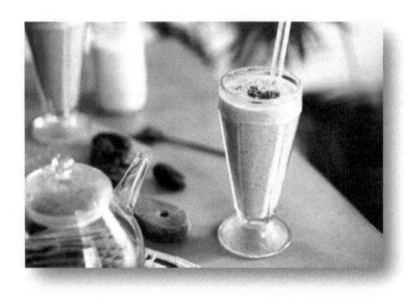

Preparation Time: 10 minutes

Cooking Time: 0 minutes

Servings: 2

Ingredients:

- 5 Medjool dates, pitted, soaked in boiling water for 5 minutes

- ¾ cup unsweetened coconut milk

- 1 teaspoon vanilla extract

- ½ teaspoon fresh lemon juice

- ¼ teaspoon sea salt, optional

- 1½ cups ice

Directions:

1. Put all the ingredients in a food processor, then blitz until it has a milkshake and smooth texture.

2. Serve immediately.

Nutrition: Calories: 380 Fat: 21.6g Carbs: 50.3g Fiber: 6.0g Protein: 3.2g

BREAD RECIPES

Mashed Potato Bread

Preparation Time: 40 minutes

Cooking Time: 2.5-3 hours

Serving Size: 2 ounces (56.7g) per slice

Ingredients:

- 2 1/3 cups bread flour

- ½ cup mashed potatoes

- One tablespoon sugar

- 1 ½ teaspoons yeast

- ¾ teaspoon salt

- ¼ cup potato water

- One tablespoon ground flax seeds

- Four teaspoons oil

Direction:

1. Put the ingredients into the pan in this order: potato water, oil, flax seeds, mashed potatoes, sugar, salt, flour, and yeast.

2. Ready the bread machine by pressing the "Basic" or "Normal" mode with a medium crust colour setting.

3. Allow the bread machine to finish all cycles.

4. Remove the bread pan from the machine.

5. Carefully take the bread from the pan.

6. Put the bread on a wire rack, then cool down before slicing.

Nutrition: Calories: 140 Carbohydrates: 26 g

Healthy Celery Loaf

Preparation Time: 2 hours 40 minutes

Cooking Time: 50 minutes

Servings: 1 loaf

Ingredients:

- 1 can (10 ounces) cream of celery soup
- tablespoons coconut milk, heated
- 1 tablespoon vegetable oil
- 1¼ teaspoons celery salt
- ¾ cup celery, fresh/sliced thin
- 1 tablespoon celery leaves, fresh, chopped
- 1 whole egg
- ¼ teaspoon sugar
- cups bread flour
- ¼ teaspoon ginger
- ½ cup quick-cooking oats
- tablespoons gluten

- teaspoons celery seeds

- 1 pack of active dry yeast

Directions:

1 Add all of the ingredients to your bread machine, carefully following the instructions of the manufacturer

2 Set the program of your bread machine to Basic/White Bread and set crust type to Medium

3 Press START

4 Wait until the cycle completes

5 Once the loaf is ready, take the bucket out and let the loaf cool for 5 minutes

6 Gently shake the bucket to remove the loaf

7 Transfer to a cooling rack, slice and serve

8 Enjoy!

Nutrition: Calories: 73 Cal Fat: 4 g Carbohydrates: 8 g Protein: 3 g Fiber: 1 g

Broccoli and Cauliflower Bread

Preparation Time: 2 hours 20 minutes

Cooking Time: 50 minutes

Servings: 1 loaf

Ingredients:

- ¼ cup water

- tablespoons olive oil

- 1 egg white

- 1 teaspoon lemon juice

- 2/3 cup grated cheddar cheese

- tablespoons green onion

- ½ cup broccoli, chopped

- ½ cup cauliflower, chopped

- ½ teaspoon lemon pepper seasoning

- cups bread flour

- 1 teaspoon bread machine yeast

Directions:

1 Add all of the ingredients to your bread machine, carefully following the instructions of the manufacturer

2 Set the program of your bread machine to Basic/White Bread and set crust type to Medium

3 Press START

4 Wait until the cycle completes

5 Once the loaf is ready, take the bucket out and let the loaf cool for 5 minutes

6 Gently shake the bucket to remove the loaf

7 Transfer to a cooling rack, slice and serve

8 Enjoy!

Nutrition: Calories: 156 Cal Fat: 8 g Carbohydrates: 17 g Protein: 5 g Fiber: 2 g

SAUCES, DRESSINGS, AND DIPS

Avocado-dill Dressing

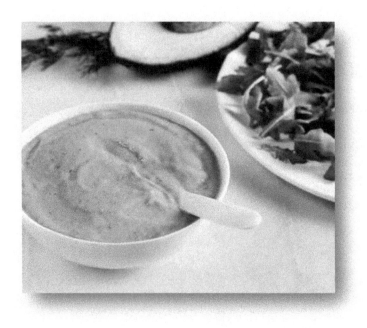

Preparation Time: 20 minutes

Cooking Time: 0 minutes

Servings: 1

Ingredients:

- 2 ounces (57 g) raw, unsalted cashews (about ½ cup)

- ½ cup water

- 3 tablespoons lemon juice

- ½ medium, ripe avocado, chopped

- 1 medium clove garlic

- 2 tablespoons chopped fresh dill

- 2 green onions, white and green parts, chopped

Directions:

1. Put the cashews, water, lemon juice, avocado, and garlic into a blender. Keep it aside for at least 15 minutes to soften the cashews.

2. Blend until everything is fully mixed. Fold in the dill and green onions, and blend briefly to retain some texture.

3. Store in an airtight container in the fridge for up to 3 days and stir well before serving.

Nutrition: Calories: 312 Fat: 21.1g Carbs: 22.6g Protein: 8.0g Fiber: 7.1g

SALADS RECIPES

Sweet Potato & Black Bean Protein Salad

Preparation Time: 15 minutes

Cooking Time: 0 minutes

Servings: 2

Ingredients:

- 1 cup dry black beans

- 4 cups of spinach

- 1 medium sweet potato

- 1 cup purple onion, chopped

- 2 tbsp. olive oil

- 2 tbsp. lime juice

- 1 tbsp. minced garlic

- ½ tbsp. chili powder

- ¼ tsp. cayenne

- ¼ cup parsley

- ¼ tsp Salt

- ¼ tsp pepper

Directions:

1. Prepare the black beans according to the method.

2. Preheat the oven to 400°F.

3. Cut the sweet potato into ¼-inch cubes and put these in a medium-sized bowl. Add the onions, 1 tablespoon of olive oil, and salt to taste.

4. Toss the ingredients until the sweet potatoes and onions are completely coated.

5. Transfer the ingredients to a baking sheet lined with parchment paper and spread them out in a single layer.

6. Put the baking sheet in the oven and roast until the sweet potatoes are starting to turn brown and crispy, around 40 minutes.

7. Meanwhile, combine the remaining olive oil, lime juice, garlic, chili powder, and cayenne thoroughly in a large bowl, until no lumps remain.

8. Remove the sweet potatoes and onions from the oven and transfer them to the large bowl.

9. Add the cooked black beans, parsley, and a pinch of salt.

10. Toss everything until well combined.

11. Then mix in the spinach, and serve in desired portions with additional salt and pepper.

12. Store or enjoy!

Nutrition: Calories 558 Total Fat 16.2g Saturated Fat 2.5g Cholesterol 0mg Sodium 390mg Total Carbohydrate 84g Dietary Fiber 20.4g Total Sugars 8.9g Protein 25.3g Vitamin D 0mcg Calcium 220mg Iron 10mg Potassium 2243mg

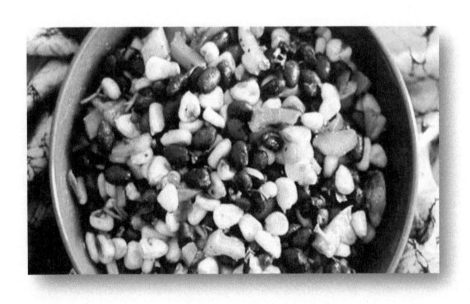

FRUIT SALAD RECIPES

Asian Fruit Salad

Preparation Time: 30 Minutes

Cooking Time: 0 Minutes

Servings: 8

Ingredients:

- Passion fruit, one-half cup (about six of the fruit)

- Papaya, one chopped

- Pineapple, one cup chunked

- Oranges, two separated into segments

- Star fruit, three sliced thin

- Mangoes, two large, peeled and chunked

- Mint, fresh, one-third cup chopped coarse

- Lime juice, one third cup

- Lime zest, one tablespoon

- Ginger, ground, one tablespoon

- Vanilla extract, one tablespoon

- Brown sugar, one half cup

- Water, four cups

Directions:

1. Mix the water and the sugar together in a medium-sized saucepan and put it over a medium to high heat until the sugar is dissolved.

2. Let this simmer for five minutes over a very low heat, so the sugar does not burn. Add in the vanilla extract and the ginger and stir well.

3. Let this cook for ten more minutes. Let the mix cool off the heat until it is room temperature, and then add in the mint, juice, and zest.

4. During the time the sauce is cooling mix together the remainder of the Ingredients in a large-sized bowl.

5. Pour the syrup mixture over the fruit in the bowl and mix gently to coat all pieces with the sauce.

6. Put the bowl in the refrigerator until the fruit is cold then serve.

Nutrition: Calories: 220 Protein: 3g Fat: 1g Carbs: 56g

ENTRÉES

Chickpea Avocado Salad Sandwiches

Preparation Time: 10 minutes

Cooking Time: 0 minutes

Servings: 4

Ingredients:

- Chickpeas, liquid drained, rinsed – 15 ounce can (1.5 cups)

- Red onion, diced - .5 cup

- Lemon juice – 2 tablespoons

- Cilantro, fresh, chopped - .25 cup

- Thyme, fresh, chopped – 1 tablespoon

- Avocado, diced – 1 cup

- Red grapes, sliced in half - .5 cup

- Celery, finely sliced - .25 cup

- Sea salt – 1 teaspoon

- Whole-wheat bread – 6 slices

Directions:

1. Place the drained and rinse chickpeas and the diced avocado in a medium-sized bowl for the purpose of mixing. Using a fork or potato masher smash the ingredients together until you form a chunky and creamy mixture. You can do this to your preference, either leaving the chickpeas mostly whole or smashing them until they are mostly creamy.

2. Add the red onion, lemon juice, fresh cilantro, fresh thyme, red grapes, celery, and sea salt to the bowl and stir all of the ingredients together until combined.

3. Divide the chickpea salad mixture between three slices of bread, and then top it off with the remaining three slices. Of course, you can always save the mixture in the fridge for another day, and then assemble your sandwiches on the day you plan to consume them. Don't fill your sandwiches with the filling more than a day ahead of time, as you don't want soggy bread.

Nutrition: Number of Calories in Individual **Servings:** 486 Protein Grams: 16 Fat Grams: 13 Total Carbohydrates Grams: 80 Net Carbohydrates Grams: 65

GRAINS AND BEANS

Veggie Paella

Preparation Time: 15 minutes

Cooking Time: 52 to 58 minutes

Servings: 4

Ingredients:

- 1 onion, coarsely chopped

- 8 medium mushrooms, sliced

- 2 small zucchinis, cut in half, then sliced ½ inch thick

- 1 leek, rinsed and sliced

- 2 large cloves garlic, crushed

- 1 medium tomato, coarsely chopped

- 3 cups low-sodium vegetable broth

- 1¼ cups long-grain brown rice

- ½ teaspoon crushed saffron threads

- Freshly ground black pepper, to taste

- ½ cup frozen green peas

- ½ cup water

- Chopped fresh parsley, for garnish

Directions:

1. Pour the water in a large wok. Add the onion and sauté for 5 minutes, or until most of the liquid is absorbed.

2. Stir in the mushrooms, zucchini, leek, and garlic and cook for 2 to 3 minutes, or until softened slightly.

3. Add the tomato, broth, rice, saffron, and pepper. Bring to a boil. Reduce the heat and simmer, covered, for 30 minutes.

4. Add the peas and continue to cook for another 5 to 10 minutes. Remove from the heat and let rest for 10 minutes to allow any excess moisture to be absorbed.

5. Sprinkle with the parsley before serving.

Nutrition: Calories: 418 Fat: 3.9g Carbs: 83.2g Protein: 12.7g Fiber: 9.2g

Spiced Tomato Brown Rice

Preparation Time: 10 minutes

Cooking Time: 15 minutes

Servings: 4 to 6

Ingredients:

- 1 onion, diced

- 1 green bell pepper, diced

- 3 cloves garlic, minced

- ¼ cup water

- 15 to 16 ounces (425 to 454g) tomatoes, chopped

- 1 tablespoon chili powder

- 2 teaspoons ground cumin

- 1 teaspoon dried basil

- ½ teaspoon Parsley Patch seasoning, general blend

- ¼ teaspoon cayenne

- 2 cups cooked brown rice

Directions:

1. Combine the onion, green pepper, garlic and water in a saucepan over medium heat. Cook for about 5 minutes, stirring constantly, or until softened.

2. Add the tomatoes and seasonings. Cook for another 5 minutes. Stir in the cooked rice. Cook for another 5 minutes to allow the flavors to blend.

3. Serve immediately.

Nutrition. Calories: 107 Fat: 1.1g Carbs: 21.1g Protein: 3.2g Fiber: 2.9g

DRINKS

Strawberry Pink Drink

Preparation Time: 10 Minutes

Cooking Time: 5 Minutes

Servings: 4

Ingredients:

- Water (1 C., Boiling)

- Sugar (2 T.)

- Acai Tea Bag (1)

- Coconut Milk (1 C.)

- Frozen Strawberries (1/2 C.)

Directions:

1. If you are looking for a little treat, this is going to be the recipe for you! You will begin by boiling your cup of water and seep the tea bag in for at least five minutes.

2. When the tea is set, add in the sugar and coconut milk. Be sure to stir well to spread the sweetness throughout the tea.

3. Finally, add in your strawberries, and you can enjoy your freshly made pink drink!

Nutrition: Calories: 321 Total Carbohydrate: 2 g Cholesterol: 13 mg Total Fat: 17 g Fiber: 2 g Protein: 9 g Sodium: 312 mg

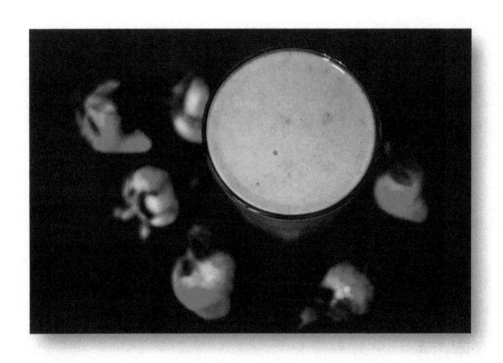

Almond Butter Brownies

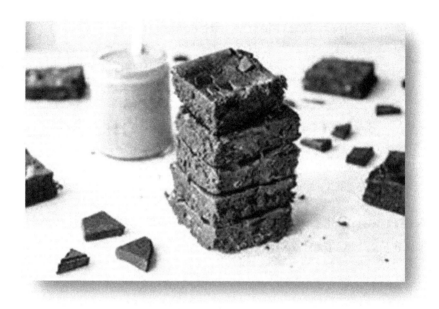

Preparation Time: 10 minutes

Cooking Time: 20 minutes

Servings: 4

Ingredients:

- 1 scoop protein powder

- 2 tbsp. cocoa powder

- 1/2 cup almond butter, melted

- 1 cup bananas, overripe

Directions:

1. Preheat the oven to 350 F/ 176 C.

1. Spray brownie tray with cooking spray.

2. Add all ingredients into the blender and blend until smooth.

3. Pour batter into the prepared dish and bake in preheated oven for 20 minutes.

4. Serve and enjoy.

Nutrition: Calories: 214 Total Carbohydrate: 2 g Cholesterol: 73 mg Total Fat: 7 g Fiber: 2g Protein: 19 g Sodium: 308 g

Quick Chocó Brownie

Preparation Time: 10 minutes

Cooking Time: 2 minutes

Servings: 1

Ingredients:

- 1/4 cup almond milk

- 1 tbsp. cocoa powder

- 1 scoop chocolate protein powder

- 1/2 tsp baking powder

Directions:

1. In a microwave-safe mug blend together baking powder, protein powder, and cocoa.

2. Add almond milk in a mug and stir well.

3. Place mug in microwave and microwave for 30 seconds.

4. Serve and enjoy.

Nutrition: Calories: 231 Total Carbohydrate: 2 g Cholesterol: 13 mg Total Fat: 15 g Fiber: 2 g Protein: 8 g Sodium: 298 mg

Coconut Peanut Butter Fudge

Preparation Time: 1 hour 15 minutes

Cooking Time: 0 minute

Servings: 20

Ingredients:

- 12 oz. smooth peanut butter

- 3 tbsp. coconut oil

- 4 tbsp. coconut cream

- 15 drops liquid stevia

- Pinch of salt

Directions:

1. Line baking tray with parchment paper.

2. Melt coconut oil in a saucepan over low heat.

3. Add peanut butter, coconut cream, stevia, and salt in a saucepan. Stir well.

4. Pour fudge mixture into the prepared baking tray and place in refrigerator for 1 hour.

5. Cut into pieces and serve.

Nutrition: Calories: 189 Total Carbohydrate: 2 g Cholesterol: 13 mg
Total Fat: 7 g Fiber: 2 g Protein: 10 g Sodium: 301 mg

DESSERTS

Cashew-Chocolate Truffles

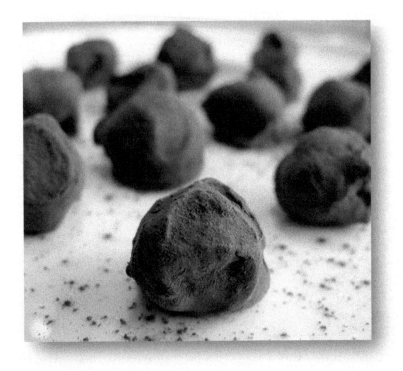

Preparation Time: 15 minutes

Cooking Time: 0 minutes

Servings: 12

Ingredients:

- 1 cup raw cashews, soaked in water overnight

- ¾ cup pitted dates

- 2 tablespoons coconut oil

- 1 cup unsweetened shredded coconut, divided

- 1 to 2 tablespoons cocoa powder, to taste

Directions:

1. Preparing the Ingredients.

2. In a food processor, combine the cashews, dates, coconut oil, ½ cup of shredded coconut, and cocoa powder. Pulse until fully incorporated; it will resemble chunky cookie dough. Spread the remaining ½ cup of shredded coconut on a plate.

3. Form the mixture into tablespoon-size balls and roll on the plate to cover with the shredded coconut. Transfer to a parchment paper–lined plate or baking sheet. Repeat to make 12 truffles.

4. Place the truffles in the refrigerator for 1 hour to set. Transfer the truffles to a storage container or freezer-safe bag and seal.

Nutrition: Calories 160 Fat 1 g Carbohydrates 1 g Sugar 0.5 g Protein 22 g Cholesterol 60 mg

Banana Chocolate Cupcakes

Preparation Time: 20 minutes

Cooking Time: 20 minutes

Servings: 1

Ingredients:

- 3 medium bananas

- 1 cup non-dairy milk

- 2 tablespoons almond butter

- 1 teaspoon apple cider vinegar

- 1 teaspoon pure vanilla extract

- 1¼ cups whole-grain flour

- ½ cup rolled oats

- ¼ cup coconut sugar (optional)

- 1 teaspoon baking powder

- ½ teaspoon baking soda

- ½ cup unsweetened cocoa powder

- ¼ cup chia seeds, or sesame seeds

- Pinch sea salt

- ¼ cup dark chocolate chips, dried cranberries, or raisins (optional)

Directions:

1. Preparing the Ingredients.

2. Preheat the oven to 350°F. Lightly grease the cups of two 6-cup muffin tins or line with paper muffin cups.

3. Put the bananas, milk, almond butter, vinegar, and vanilla in a blender and purée until smooth. Or stir together in a large bowl until smooth and creamy.

4. Put the flour, oats, sugar (if using), baking powder, baking soda, cocoa powder, chia seeds, salt, and chocolate chips in another large bowl, and stir to combine. Mix together the wet and dry ingredients, stirring as little as possible. Spoon into muffin cups, and bake for 20 to 25 minutes. Take the cupcakes out of the oven and let them cool fully before taking out of the muffin tins, since they'll be very moist.

Nutrition: Calories 295 Fat 17 g Carbohydrates 4 g Sugar 0.1 g Protein 29 g Cholesterol 260 mg

Minty Fruit Salad

Preparation Time: 15 minutes

Cooking Time: 5 minutes

Servings: 4

Ingredients:

- ¼ cup lemon juice (about 2 small lemons)

- 4 teaspoons maple syrup or agave syrup

- 2 cups chopped pineapple

- 2 cups chopped strawberries

- 2 cups raspberries

- 1 cup blueberries

- 8 fresh mint leaves

Directions:

Preparing the Ingredients.

1. Beginning with 1 mason jar, add the ingredients in this order:

2. 1 tablespoon of lemon juice, 1 teaspoon of maple syrup, ½ cup of pineapple, ½ cup of strawberries, ½ cup of raspberries, ¼ cup of blueberries, and 2 mint leaves.

3. Repeat to fill 3 more jars. Close the jars tightly with lids.

4. Place the airtight jars in the refrigerator for up to 3 days.

Nutrition: Calories 339 Fat 17.5 g Carbohydrates 2 g Sugar 2 g Protein 44 g Cholesterol 100 mg

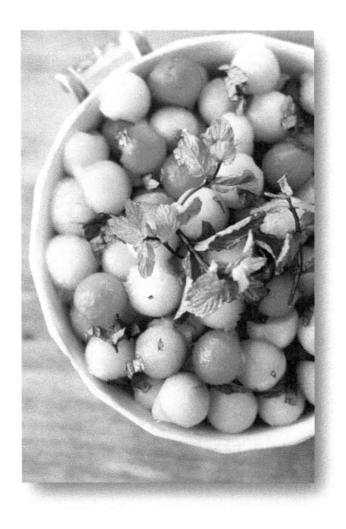

Cherry-Vanilla Rice Pudding (Pressure cooker)

Preparation Time: 5 minutes

Cooking Time: 30 minutes

Servings: 4-6

Ingredients:

- 1 cup short-grain brown rice

- 1¾ cups nondairy milk, plus more as needed

- 1½ cups water

- 4 tablespoons unrefined sugar or pure maple syrup (use 2 tablespoons if you use a sweetened milk), plus more as needed

- 1 teaspoon vanilla extract (use ½ teaspoon if you use vanilla milk)

- Pinch salt

- ¼ cup dried cherries or ½ cup fresh or frozen pitted cherries

Directions:

1.   Preparing the Ingredients. In your electric pressure cooker's cooking pot, combine the rice, milk, water, sugar, vanilla, and salt.

2.   High pressure for 30 minutes. Close and lock the lid, and select High Pressure for 30 minutes.

3.   Pressure Release. Once the **Cooking Time:** is complete, let the pressure release naturally, about 20 minutes. Unlock and remove the lid. Stir in the cherries and put the lid back on loosely for about 10 minutes. Serve, adding more milk or sugar, as desired.

Nutrition: Calories 420 Fat 27.4 g Carbohydrates 2 g Sugar 0.3 g Protein 46.3 g Cholesterol 98 mg

OTHER RECIPES

Delicious Lentil Soup

Preparation Time: 15 Minutes

Cooking Time: 25 Minutes

Servings: 4

Ingredients:

- 1 tbsp. Olive Oil

- 4 cups Vegetable Stock

- 1 Onion, finely chopped

- 2 Carrots, medium

- 1 cup Lentils, dried

- 1 tsp. Cumin

Directions:

1. To make this healthy soup, first, you need to heat the oil in a medium-sized skillet over medium heat.

2. Once the oil becomes hot, stir in the cumin and then the onions.

3. Sauté those for 3 minutes or until the onion is slightly transparent and cooked.

4. To this, add the carrots and toss them well.

5. Next, stir in the lentils. Mix well.

6. Now, pour in the vegetable stock and give a good stir until everything comes together.

7. As the soup mixture starts to boil, reduce the heat and allow it to simmer for 10 minutes while keeping the pan covered.

8. Turn off the heat and then transfer the mixture to a bowl.

9. Finally, blend it with an immersion blender or in a high-speed blender for 1 minute or until you get a rich, smooth mixture.

10. Serve it hot and enjoy.

Nutrition: Calories: 251 Kcal Protein: 14g Carbohydrates: 41.3g Fat: 4.1g

Trail Mix

Preparation Time: 10 Minutes

Cooking Time: 10 Minutes

Servings: 2

Ingredients:

- 1 cup Walnuts, raw

- 2 cups Tart Cherries, dried

- 1 cup Pumpkin Seeds, raw

- 1 cup Almonds, raw

- ½ cup Vegan Dark Chocolate

- 1 cup Cashew

Directions:

1. First, mix all the ingredients needed to make the trail mix in a large mixing bowl until combined well.

2. Store in an air-tight container.

Nutrition: Calories: 596 Kcal Protein: 17.5g Carbohydrates: 46.1g Fat: 39.5g

Flax Crackers

Preparation Time: 5 Minutes

Cooking Time: 60 Minutes

Servings: 4 to 6

Ingredients:

- 1 cup Flaxseeds, whole

- 2 cups Water

- ¾ cup Flaxseeds, grounded

- 1 tsp. Sea Salt

- ½ cup Chia Seeds

- 1 tsp. Black Pepper

- ½ cup Sunflower Seeds

Directions:

1. Using a large bowl, you need to put all your ingredients then mix them well. Soak them in a water for about 10 to 15 minutes.

2. After that, transfer the mixture to a parchment paper-lined baking sheet and spread it evenly. Tip: Make sure the paper lines the edges as well.

3. Next, bake it for 60 minutes at 350 °F.

4. Once the time is up, flip the entire bar and take off the parchment paper.

5. Bake for half an hour or until it becomes crispy and browned.

6. Allow it to cool completely and then break it down.

Nutrition: Calories: 251cal Proteins: 9.2g Carbohydrates: 14.9g Fat: 16g

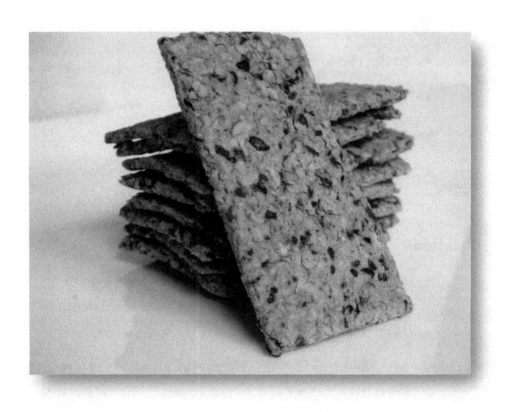

CPSIA information can be obtained
at www.ICGtesting.com
Printed in the USA
BVHW090038090621
609009BV00009B/1236